The 2005 Pfizer Medical School Manual

A Practical Guide To Getting Into Medical School

Mike Magee, M.D.

The 2005 Pfizer Medical School Manual/Mike Magee, M.D.
104 p.   1 cm.
ISBN: 1-889793-15-9
Printed in Canada

The 2005 Pfizer Medical School Manual
is provided as part of the
Pfizer Medical Humanities Initiative,
a program which encourages
the development of humanistically
and scientifically balanced
physicians committed to
patients, families, and
their communities.

For more information about the
Pfizer Medical Humanities Initiative,
contact:
http://www.positiveprofiles.com

Table of Contents

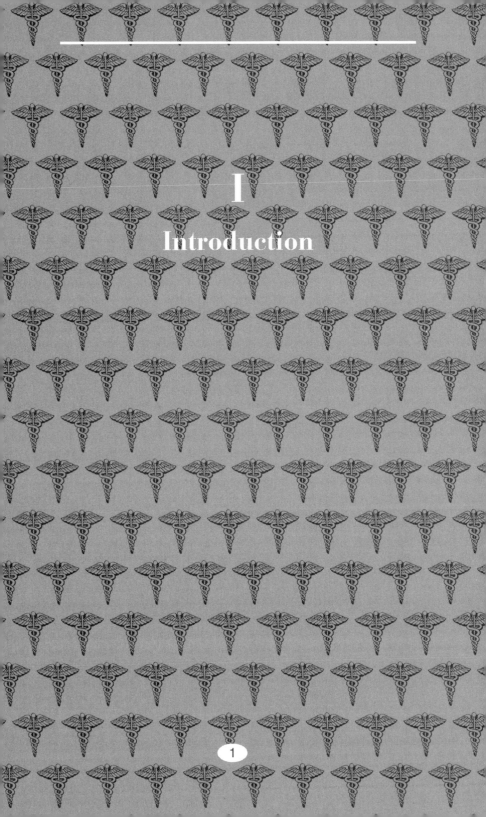

I
Introduction

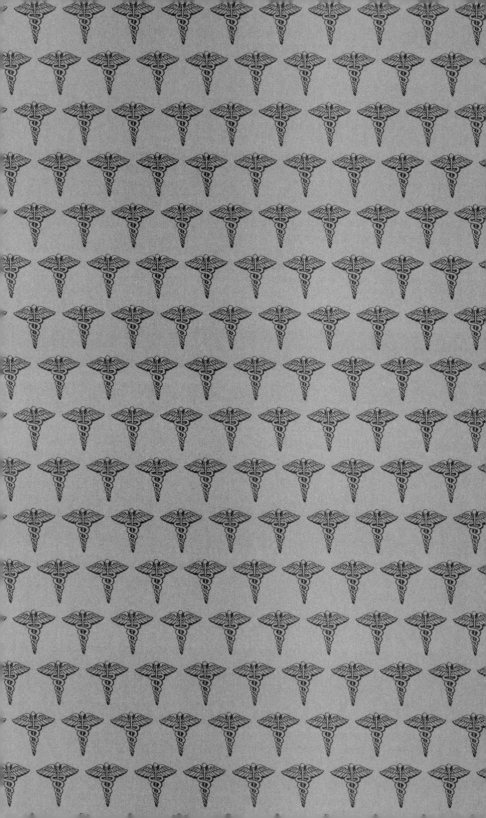

An Introductory Message by Author Mike Magee, M.D.

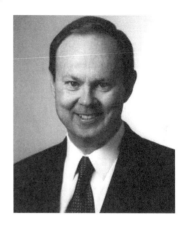

*T*his book is dedicated to those who seek to devote their lives to a career in medicine. It is intended to assist would-be physicians as they navigate the complex and often daunting medical school admissions process.

In an era that heralds accelerated breakthroughs and scientific discoveries, medical science is on the brink of an unprecedented ability to understand and manipulate human life. Our understanding of the genetic and molecular mechanisms underlying diseases has greatly expanded the scope of the possible. Knowledge of the genome will allow us to predict and prevent diseases before they start. Future physicians can anticipate a constant stream of newly minted medical advances to revolutionize their medical practice, particularly the treatment of heart disease, arthritis, diabetes, Alzheimer's and cancer.

Physicians who thoughtfully and passionately embrace this medical and technological revolution will shape the future of medicine. Medicine will also be shaped by demographic changes. By 2030, 50% of American adults will be 50 or more years old, and the population of adults over 85 years old will have doubled. The challenge of meeting the ever-increasing demand for quality health care will depend upon progress in scientific understanding.

Through all the medical breakthroughs and demographic changes to come, our need for interpersonal connection will remain. Medicine will always be a profession that marries the role of medical mystery solver with compassionate healer. Medical schools will forever seek students who communicate effectively, who rigorously pursue intellectual excellence, and who find purpose, satisfaction and dignity in human service.

This book is not a secret formula that will guarantee admission to medical school. It does provide aspiring physicians with specific, practical recommendations that will help them positively and memorably present themselves to prospective medical schools. With a call to those committed to transforming their knowledge of health and science into actions that will improve people's lives, and with wholehearted endorsement of your career choice, I urge tomorrow's physicians onward!

Sincerely,

Mike Magee ms

Mike Magee, M.D.
Host, Health Politics
www.healthpolitics.com

II
Overview

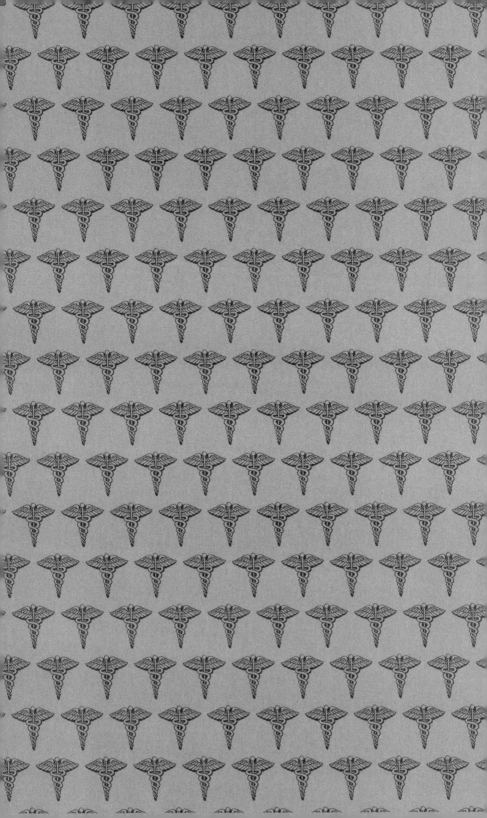

II Overview

There are approximately 80,000 students at any one time enrolled in America's 145 medical schools. Each year this unique body of talented and diverse individuals is revitalized with approximately 20,618 women and men chosen from more than 41,926 applicants. These medical students are highly qualified, having fulfilled exacting science requirements and achieved excellent grade point averages and MCAT scores.

With more than twice as many applicants as there are seats, how do medical schools decide whom to accept? Four criteria are used to evaluate applicants:
• Grade point average,
• MCAT scores,
• Letters of recommendation,
• Interviews, are often the determining factor in accepting or rejecting candidates.

As important as the interview is, preparation for it is often overlooked. The rigorous undergraduate science curriculum, the demanding process of choosing and applying to schools, the hours of study for MCAT exams, and the development of relationships with professors who will write insightful, personal letters of recommendation often take precedence over preparation for an admissions interview. Yet, successful interviews require research, introspection and analytical thought. Chapter IV of this manual prepares applicants for medical school interviews.

Undergraduate Preparation

Today, medical schools accept a broad range of undergraduate majors. Indeed, approximately 15% of applicants for the allopathic medical school Class of 2007 (who entered medical school in Fall, 2003) majored in humanities and social sciences. The acceptance rate for liberal arts majors roughly mirrored the overall acceptance rate. Still, most applicants choose a traditional path, with approximately 81% of the allopathic medical school Class of 2007 majoring in biological or physical sciences.

Most colleges and universities maintain a pre-medical advisory office. While advice on curricular choices varies from school to school, undergraduates should enroll in courses that will develop their competence in required sciences as well as contribute to their well-rounded candidacy.

Most medical schools require successful completion of the following laboratory courses:
- introductory biology (one year)
- inorganic or general chemistry (one year)
- organic chemistry (one year)
- physics (one year)

Other courses commonly required include:
- calculus or college math or statistics
- English (one year)
- humanities electives

- anatomy and physiology
- biochemistry
- genetics

Since the MCAT test required for admission to medical school assesses your knowledge of science concepts and principles, as well as problem-solving, critical thinking and writing skills, complete these courses during the first three years of college so that by your junior year you can take the April or August MCATs.

Allopathic vs. Osteopathic Medical Schools

In the United States and its territories, 125 allopathic medical schools grant Doctorates of Medicine, or M.D.s, and 20 osteopathic medical schools grant Doctorates of Osteopathy, or D.O.s.

The first school of medicine in the United States was founded at the University of Pennsylvania in 1765 by John Morgan, a young surgeon. In 1892, some 127 years later, Andrew Taylor Still, M.D., founded the first School of Osteopathic Medicine in Missouri. This school emphasized musculoskeletal training and manipulation to aid bodily function. Though chartered by state law to grant graduates an M.D., Taylor chose instead to grant Doctorates of Osteopathy, or D.O.s.

Over the next century, the two branches of medicine often clashed. By 1974, the federal and state government as well as the American Medical Association recognized both M.D.s and D.O.s as legally separate but equal branches of medicine. Today, allopathic and osteopathic medical schools share the following characteristics:

- Applicants possess four-year undergraduate degrees and meet similar science prerequisites
- Accepted students must complete four years of medical school, including two years of didactic and two years of clinical experience
- Graduates may pursue specialist or generalist tracks
- Graduates must pass board exams for licensure
- Graduates are qualified to commence residency training programs in fully accredited hospitals

To learn how students enrolled in allopathic schools compared to those enrolled in osteopathic schools, see Chapter V, pages 55-56. To learn more about allopathic medical schools, contact the Association of American Medical Colleges at www.aamc.org. For osteopathic medical schools, contact the American Association of Colleges of Osteopathic Medicine at www.aacom.org.

Application to Medical School

One hundred eighteen schools and programs of the 125 allopathic medical schools participate in the American Medical College Application Service, or AMCAS, for the 2005 entering class. The AMCAS www.aamc.org/amcas electronic application is available on the web in April of each year. AMCAS processes and forwards your application and MCAT scores to the individual schools to which you apply beginning around June 1st. Application through AMCAS allows you to complete the application process once and to simultaneously apply to any of the 118 participating allopathic schools and programs. The seven allopathic medical schools that do not participate in AMCAS are noted below:

- University of Missouri-Kansas City School of Medicine
- University of North Dakota School of Medicine and Health Sciences
- Texas A&M University System Health Science Center College of Medicine
- Texas Tech University Health Sciences Center School of Medicine
- University of Texas Medical School at Galveston
- University of Texas Medical School at Houston
- University of Texas Medical School at San Antonio

The AMCAS application fee is based upon the number of schools to which applicants apply. The fee for an application is $160 for the first school and $30.00 for each additional school regardless of the point at which you add school designations. In addition to this fee, individual medical schools have supplemental application fees that range from $25 to $100. Upon receipt of your AMCAS application, each school usually sends secondary application materials as well as a bill for the school's individual application fee. Failure to remit this fee may result in no further action being taken on your application.

To obtain an AMCAS web application (the paper version is no longer produced) or additional information about AMCAS, contact:

AMCAS
American Medical College Application Service
Section for Student Services
2501 M Street, NW, Lobby-26
Washington, DC 20037-1300
(202) 828-0600
www.aamc.org

All osteopathic medical schools participate in a comparable application service. The American Association of Colleges of Osteopathic Medicine Application Service, or AACOMAS, processes and forwards your application and MCAT scores to the individual schools to which you apply beginning around June 1st.

To obtain an AACOMAS application, available in April, contact your college advisory office, AACOMAS participating schools, or AACOMAS at:

AACOMAS
American Association of Colleges of Osteopathic Medicine Application Service
5550 Friendship Blvd.
Suite 310
Chevy Chase, MD 20815
(301) 968-4190
www.aacom.org

The MCAT

The MCAT is a standardized multiple choice and written examination administered semi-annually, on an April Saturday and on an August Saturday. Most schools recommend that the test, which is required for admission to medical school, be taken 12-18 months prior to intended enrollment. An April MCAT is recommended so that results are ready in time for your AMCAS and/or AACOMAS applications. While you may repeat the test, it is unwise to take MCATs "just for practice" because all MCAT scores are recorded on your application. It is best to do well on your first take.

The MCAT assesses problem-solving, critical thinking, writing skills and knowledge of science concepts and principles prerequisite to the study of medicine. The four components of the MCAT are:

- Verbal Reasoning, 60 questions, 85 minutes, a test of reading comprehension, reasoning skills and critical thought. Content is drawn from humanities, social sciences and natural sciences.

- Biological Sciences, 77 questions, 100 minutes, a test of general biology concepts and problem-solving skills that includes graphs, tables and charts.

- Physical Sciences, 77 questions, 100 minutes, a test of physics, organic and inorganic chemistry, DNA and genetics concepts and problem-solving skills that includes graphs, tables and charts.

- Writing Sample, two essay questions, 60 minutes, a test of writing and analytical skills.

Four scores are reported, one for each section. Verbal Reasoning, Physical Sciences and Biological Sciences grades are scored on a scale from 1 (lowest) to 15 (highest). The Writing Sample is scored on a scale ranging from J (lowest) to T (highest).

Information and registration for the April MCAT exam are generally available in February and can be found at www.aamc.org/mcat. Registration for the MCAT is only available online.

Payment of approximately $190 covers administration of the MCAT exam and release of your test scores to AMCAS participating schools and 8 non-AMCAS participating schools. The $190 MCAT fee may be reduced or waived. Waiver materials can be found at www.aamc.org/fap.

In addition to test preparation texts such as Arco's, Flower's, Baron's, Monarch's and Barnes and Noble's, students may find the following resources useful in preparing for the MCAT:

1. Association of American Medical Colleges
    MCAT Publication – Student Manual
    Membership and Publication Orders
    2450 N Street, NW
    Washington, DC 20037-1129
    (202) 828-0416
    www.aamc.org
    AAMC provides a student manual of sample tests.

2. Kaplan Educational Centers
   131 West 56th Street
   New York, NY 10019
   (800) KAP-TEST
   www.kaplan.com
   An MCAT review course is available.

3. Princeton Review
   2315 Broadway
   New York, NY 10024
   (212) 925-6447
   www.review.com
   An MCAT review course is available.

Early Decision Program

Two-thirds of American medical schools participate in an Early Decision Program for highly qualified applicants with a strong preference for one school. Students who participate in this program agree to apply to no other school prior to the medical college's October 1 decision. Students agree to enroll in the early decision school if accepted. Students not accepted early decision may be deferred for consideration with regular candidates, or rejected.

One disadvantage of the EDP is that it prevents application to other schools until after October 1st. This delay can significantly decrease your chances of admission compared to an application submitted earlier in the cycle. In 2003, 55% of the allopathic candidates received acceptances compared to 49% of the general applicant pool. This is lower than the prior year's 70% acceptance rate for EDP candidates.

Recommended Number of Applications

For the Class of 2007, students applying to allopathic medical schools submitted an average of 11.3 applications. Students applying to osteopathic medical schools submitted applications to an average of 5.49 medical schools.

The data indicates little difference in acceptance rates for those applying to multiple schools. In 2003, of those who applied to seven to nineteen allopathic schools, 53% were accepted by at least one school, while those who applied to more than nineteen schools had an acceptance rate of 59%. More important than acceptance rates is choosing schools that match your specific qualifications and interests, and that have historically accepted students from your college.

A number of factors may enhance your chances for admission. These include state residency, institutions where you apply early decision or have an existing personal connection, and membership in a special interest group.

Selecting a Medical School

To decide upon a medical school, read available literature both from and about different schools, visit campuses and their web sites, and discuss schools with your advisors and with current medical students. 10 factors to consider when comparing schools are:

1. Policies favoring state residents
2. Size of student body
3. Student:faculty ratio
4. Patient care opportunities
5. Geographic location
6. Student services
7. Sources of financial support
8. Cost
9. Unique volunteer/research/leadership activities
10. Positioning for residencies or future graduate studies

Differences in curriculum should also be noted. 10 curricular areas expanding in American medical schools are:

1. Nutrition
2. Geriatrics
3. Epidemiology
4. Environmental health
5. Preventive and community health care
6. Medical humanities
7. Medical ethics

8. Clinical decision making

9. Medical information systems

10. Socioeconomics of medicine

Chances for admission may be enhanced if the following characteristics apply to you:

1. State resident

2. Member of a under-served group

3. Willingness to practice in under-served or rural areas

4. Plans to become a primary care physician

5. Existing relationship with school

6. Residence in adjacent, contractually linked states

7. Early submission of application

8. Your college is one of the medical school's "feeder" schools

9. Credentials comparable to or exceeding the school's applicant pool

III

The Application Process

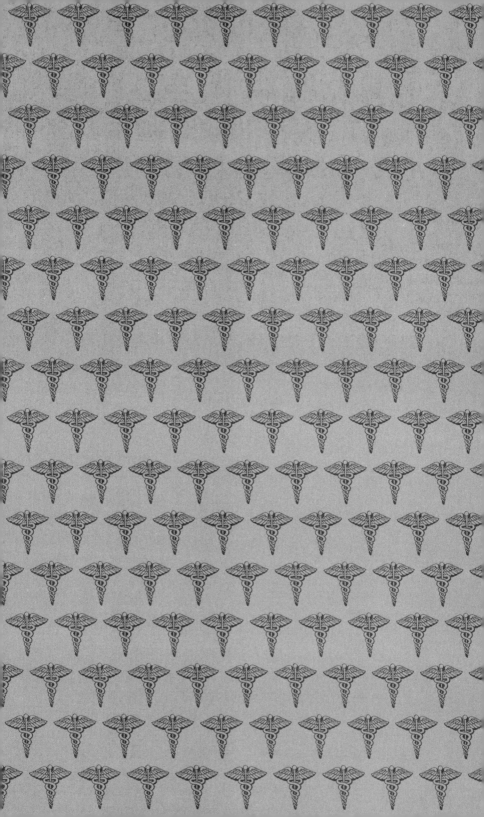

III The Application Process

Calendar of Deadlines

Entering Medical School in 2006

MCAT Review/Applications	January, 2005
April MCAT Registration	January 2005
April MCAT Registration Deadline	March 11, 2005
AMCAS Begins Accepting Official Transcripts	May/ or anytime after application is available
AACOMAS Begins Accepting Official Transcripts	April, 2005
April MCAT Administered	April 16, 2004
AACOMAS Paper and Web Application Available	May, 2005
AMCAS Web Application Available	May, 2005
AMCAS Submissions Begin	June, 2005
AACOMAS Submissions Begin	Anytime after application is available
April MCAT Results Available	June, 2005
August MCAT Registration Deadline	July 15, 2005
Optimal Submission of Complete Application	June, 2005
Early Decision Program Application Filed	August 2, 2005
Early Decision Application Complete	August 2, 2005
August MCAT Administered	August 20, 2005
Early Decision Rendered	October 1, 2005
August MCAT Results Available	October, 2005
Application Deadline for Most Medical Schools	October 15 or November 1, 2005

Timeline

Create a timeline by first deciding when you want to enter medical school. Then, in sequential order, follow these steps:

1. Fulfill science requirements

Basic undergraduate sciences in biology, chemistry and physics, including laboratories, are a prerequisite for application to medical school. To be competitive, you should attain A's and B's in these courses. By January of your junior year, request and verify the accuracy of transcripts from all colleges attended.

2. Volunteer or work in health settings

Most medical schools seek prospective students who have been exposed to physicians and patients in health-related settings. Such experience demonstrates your knowledge and commitment to health science and to human service. Interviews often aggressively explore just how significant your involvement was.

3. Broaden your course selection

If possible, take classes that will expand your potential as a caring individual, community leader and physician.

4. Develop onsite advisors

Cultivate strong relationships with faculty who can advise and support you. These relationships will surely enrich your academic experience.

Professors can recommend courses and appropriate medical schools and write letters of recommendation. Professors might also invite you to work with them on projects or in their labs. Meet with professors and advisors at least twice each semester to discuss your aspirations, intellectual passions and extracurricular activities.

5. Prepare for the MCAT

Generally, performance on the MCAT mirrors SAT performance. Home study programs or more formalized MCAT review courses can improve performance.

6. Take the April MCAT if possible

The MCAT exam is offered twice each year, in April and August. An April MCAT allows scores to be delivered to AMCAS or AACOMAS in time for AMCAS and AACOMAS applications and affords the opportunity to repeat the test if necessary. The test should be taken 12-18 months prior to intended enrollment. For more information, contact MCAT at (319) 337-1357 or www.aamc.org.

7. Submit transcripts to AMCAS/AACOMAS

Transcripts require the greatest lead-time and should be requested, verified and sent prior to completion of your AMCAS, non-AMCAS or AACOMAS applications. Since official transcripts are accepted by AMCAS, AACOMAS and non-AMCAS schools beginning in mid March, you should request that each school you have attended send you a transcript.

Check each transcript for accuracy and then ask each school to send a single, official transcript to AMCAS or AACOMAS and an official transcript to each of your non-AMCAS participating schools.

Applications for AMCAS and AACOMAS are generally available in May and submissions begin around June1. For information regarding application to allopathic medical schools, contact AMCAS at (202) 828-0600 or www.aamc.org. Application information regarding non-AMCAS schools must be obtained directly from these schools. For information regarding application to osteopathic medical schools, contact AACOMAS at (301) 968-4190 or www.aacom.org.

8. Submit applications early to optimize your chances

Early applications are associated with higher acceptance rates and greater likelihood of being invited for interviews. Submit applications as soon as possible and include your scores, transcripts, personal essay and letters of recommendation. Maintain records of all your applications.

9. Monitor application submission

Track the arrival of your applications to ensure their completeness and their receipt by each school to which you are applying. To assume safe delivery is to court disappointment. You must be your own best advocate in the application process.

The Admissions Committee and Its Function

In most medical schools, the Admissions Committee is comprised of 15 or more members of the general faculty, as well as representatives from the medical student body. The Dean of Admissions usually chairs the committee and he or she reports directly to the Medical School Dean. The committee first evaluates students by reviewing their credentials and letters of recommendation. Committee members also conduct interviews and submit written evaluations of interviewees. The entire committee discusses each candidate's application, with the interviewer often commenting on his or her impressions. During committee meetings, all members evaluate interviewed students and participate in the voting. Meetings are usually held weekly from early fall through the end of spring.

The File

The Admissions Office maintains a file on each applicant. This file includes your AMCAS, AACOMAS, or non-AMCAS school application, your science and non-science GPA, grades from all transcripts, a list of the schools you have attended, all MCAT scores, letters of recommendation and your personal statement. In addition, your file may contain notations of support, and records of all written, verbal, and onsite inquiries you have made regarding your admission to the school.

The Personal Essay

The personal essay is the only truly personal statement you make prior to your interview. Use the essay to sell yourself. An effective essay will distinguish you from all other candidates, most of whom will have credentials nearly identical to your own. Some counsel:

Do

1. Catch the reader's attention from your first sentence. Skilled journalists know the power of a short, compelling lead. Keep your reader's attention with a well-organized, concise personal essay. A strong close will further convince your audience that it is in their best interest to interview you.

2. Describe specific accomplishments, giving the reader a well-focused and articulate view of who you are, your interests, experience and history.

3. In presenting your many achievements, do so within the context of gratitude for the opportunity rather than as a testimonial to your greatness or conquests.

4. Explain information in your application that might be viewed negatively by an admissions committee. This includes course failures, withdrawals, low MCAT scores, or other issues that might detract from your strength as an applicant.

5. Focus on honest, concrete, original, biographical information. Use your own voice. If you do quote someone, make sure the quote is highly relevant and invigorates your message. Hackneyed quotes, no; fresh, witty, wise and pertinent, yes.

6. Make your essay visually inviting to read. Revise carefully for correct punctuation, spelling and grammar. Have others critique the essay for accuracy, clarity and style.

Don't

1. Criticize your school, departments or teachers. Stay positive.

2. Discuss controversial or argumentative views. Sell yourself.

3. Try to make too many points. You have one page to convey two to three messages. Provide evidence that will convince your reader that you are a winning candidate who will make the school and the reader proud. Lead the reader to this conclusion but don't state this conclusion yourself.

Transcripts

AMCAS and AACOMAS will provide you with a Transcript Matching Form. Obtain copies of transcripts for all undergraduate schools you have attended by January of your junior year. Once you have checked these for accuracy, have the registrars send official transcripts to AMCAS, AACOMAS and non-AMCAS schools. Complete the Academic Record portion of your AMCAS, AACOMAS or non-AMCAS application and send the application. Note that the Transcript Matching Form must accompany each transcript.

Chronology

1. Request and verify accuracy of transcripts from all schools attended.

2. Have each college send official transcripts and send Transcript Matching Forms to AMCAS, AACOMAS and non-AMCAS medical schools.

3. Expect notification of receipt of transcripts from AMCAS, AACOMAS and non-AMCAS medical schools two to three weeks after requesting that these be sent.

4. Obtain AMCAS, AACOMAS and non-AMCAS application forms.

5. Complete and copy forms for your records.

6. Send completed AMCAS, AACOMAS and non-AMCAS application forms with fees.

7. Expect notification of receipt of your application from AMCAS, AACOMAS and non-AMCAS medical schools two to three weeks after you send these.

8. Pay individual medical schools' requested supplemental application fees.

9. Send mid-year grades directly to schools.

The Purpose of the Interview

The interview provides the medical school with an opportunity to learn more about applicants. It also allows the medical school to promote its own unique features. By its nature, the interview is primarily subjective. It provides useful information that actively supplements the objective information in your application.

In most cases, the interview is structured to be non-confrontational, supportive and open. Most experienced interviewers concentrate on lowering the stress level rather than raising it, and expect the applicants to be relaxed and to be themselves. Within this open setting, the applicants are provided enough time to thoughtfully answer questions.

The institution seeks women and men with outstanding intellectual and personal qualifications. The admissions committee works to select a group of individuals who are diverse in backgrounds, training and talents, yet will function well together as a class.

Interviews help the committee identify a cohesive group of highly qualified individuals.

Qualifications Evaluated

Objective (GPA, MCAT) and subjective (recommendations, personal essay, interview) criteria help the admissions committee evaluate your application. These objective and subjective tools reveal your:

1. Personality
2. Maturity and honesty
3. Interpersonal skills
4. Communication skills
5. Motivation and commitment to practice medicine
6. Leadership qualities
7. Humanistic, social, and ethical concerns
8. Depth and breadth of knowledge
9. Critical thinking and coping skills
10. Creativity and original thinking

Committee Assessment

Generally, the interviewer is asked to prepare a report as soon as possible after the interview. Most evaluations are written in the interviewer's narrative style. The interviewer is asked to create a synopsis of the interview with his or her impressions. Often, the report will include interesting highlights that have been gleaned from the application folder. Most institutions grade interviews and merge interview scores with scores for MCATs, GPA, and letters of recommendation. The summation of these four scores creates a composite score. Then, candidates are ranked as outstanding, excellent, very good, good or average.

A formal presentation of the candidate before the entire committee occurs a week or two after the interview. Objective scores of GPA, both science and non-science, MCATs, and grades for letters of recommendation and interviews are presented to the committee. The interviewer is often asked to summarize the candidate and he or she uses this opportunity to promote the student's candidacy, reinforcing unique strengths and providing explanation for any weaknesses in the application. A full discussion ensues with questions directed to the interviewer. Finally, a consensus is reached as to whether the applicant should be accepted or denied admission.

Protocol for Tracking Status of Application

Medical schools emphasize the integrity of the admissions process. The interviewer acts as an agent of the committee, and the decision whether to admit an applicant is a committee decision. All inquiries and communications that follow your interview should be directed to the admissions office. Do not attempt to contact the interviewer or Dean of Admissions directly or through agents for yourself. The Dean of Admissions will contact you when a decision is made.

One caveat: often students withhold all communications with the admissions office for fear of "bothering them." In some medical schools, the number of oral and written contacts with the admissions office are tracked as a reflection of your interest. You should always write the Dean of Admissions and your interviewer a thank you note following your interview. You may also check the status of your application from time to time and express your continued interest in the school.

10 Common Mistakes

1. Inadequate preparation for MCAT exams
MCAT performance mirrors SAT performance. If you are an average standardized test taker, consider an MCAT review course.

2. Late application
Submit applications early. This requires excellent planning and coordination of transcripts, MCAT's, recommendations, and applications. Ideally, you should begin planning two years before you intend to enroll.

3. Poor performance in core sciences
To be competitive, A's and B's in core science

courses are generally required. An occasional C gets by, especially if accompanied by excellent MCAT's. Repeat core courses where you earned a C or below to demonstrate your mastery of the subject matter.

4. Lack of volunteer or health service experience

It has become a general expectation that candidates will pursue experiences that demonstrate growth as a caring, service-oriented individual in the field of health care. This experience exposes your understanding, and commitment to, a life of medicine.

5. Poor choice of references

A single poor reference, even subtly stated, can send an application off track. Nurture relationships with future references early. Carefully assess the level of an individual's support for you. Consider choosing those who have already demonstrated concrete support for you through grades or other forms of recognition.

6. Poor personal essay

Write a clear, concise, well-organized and interesting statement. Check its grammar, punctuation, spelling and clarity. Seek qualified or expert critique and revise accordingly.

7. Failure to monitor application status

The application process is complex and requires sequential coordinated actions. Ensure that your completed application materials are submitted and confirm their receipt by July or August.

8. Inadequate research of school

Some of the 145 medical schools will ideally suit your personality, interests and talents; others will not. Thoroughly research medical colleges by reviewing literature, visiting campuses and conferring with pre-medical advisers, alumni and current medical students. Also consider factors such as in-state versus out-of-state admission rates.

9. Inadequate preparation for your interview

Although the interview commonly carries a quarter of the decision weight, and can actually collapse an otherwise qualified applicant, many students continue to "wing it." Careful research, preparation and performance are a must. The cardinal sins: appearing arrogant or disinterested.

10. Lack of post-interview follow through

In some schools, all verbal, written and physical contacts are captured in your application file. A thank you note to the Dean of Admissions and your interviewer is always appreciated. Gratitude is a becoming attitude in everyone, and a thank you letter leaves a favorable impression on the people who may accept you. Occasional respectful contacts to check on the status of your application are generally received as an expression of continued interest.

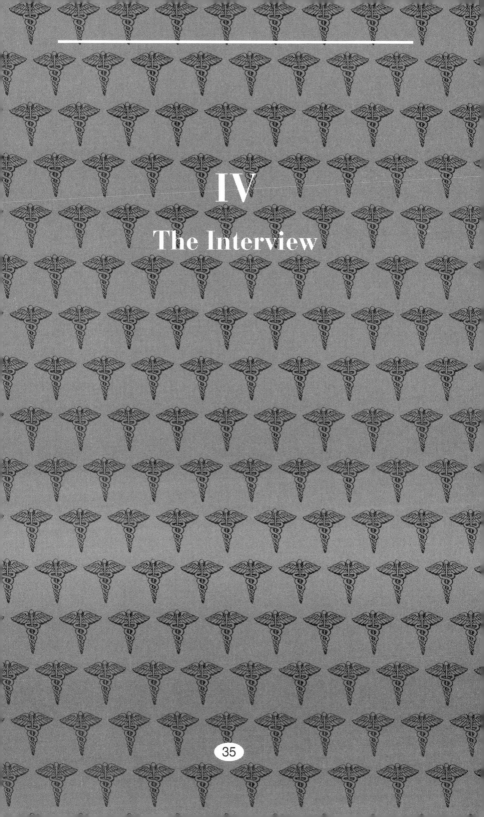

IV
The Interview

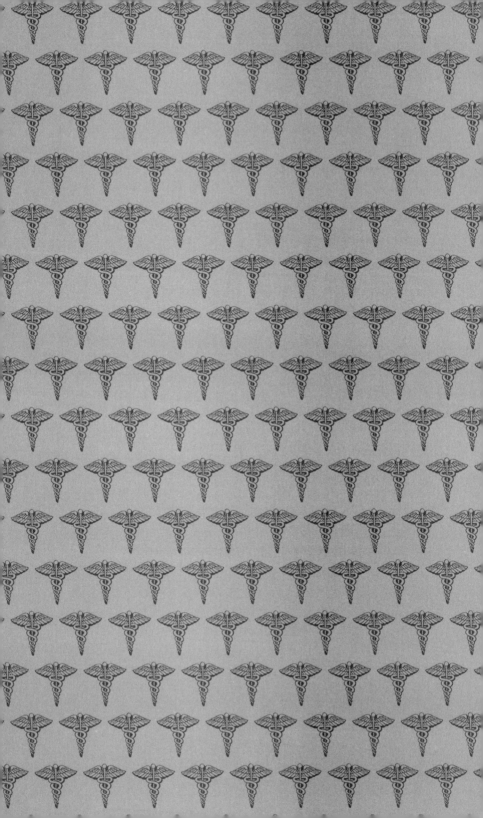

IV   The Interview

A Familiar Format

The most frequent type of interaction between two individuals is an interview with one individual soliciting information and the other providing it. Regard the medical school interview as an exchange of information. Since you were young, you have been approached and have approached others to obtain information. An interview also allows people to develop a relationship and form an impression of one other. The interview is a most flexible format that can be highly individualized. It can move forward in a prearranged manner or adapt and pursue unexpected lines of inquiry. Thorough preparation allows you to take advantage of this format. Be prepared to provide accurate and comprehensive information while keeping it positive.

Preparation for the Interview

To assure a successful interview, prepare. Think of yourself as a reporter assigned an important issue to investigate. You need a clear understanding of the organization and individuals who will be interviewing you, and the message and image you intend to convey. Review the school's catalogue and other sources of information.

1. **Conduct the following self-inventory before your interview:**
- What is your objective?
- What is your message and how does it support your objective?
- Who is your audience?
- What do you know about this institution, its people, its curriculum and its culture?
- What do they know about you?
- Have you reviewed your own application?
- What within your application makes you uncomfortable?
- What do you hope they won't ask you and how will you answer when they do?
- Where and when is the interview?
- Have you made adequate arrangements for lodging?
- Have you allotted extra time so that you can arrive at your interview relaxed and on time?

2. **Interview Questions to Expect**
   Here are questions commonly asked during medical school interviews. Be prepared to answer each:
- What do you believe in?
- What do you care about?
- How does that caring express itself?
- How did you investigate a career in medicine?
- What made you decide to pursue a career in medicine?
- What is your favorite type of teaching style?
- What branch of medicine most interests you?

- Who knows you the best in this world?
- How would that person describe you, and what advice have they provided you?
- What teamwork experiences have you had?
- Who are your heroes?
- What are your strengths and weaknesses?
- What skills have you developed outside the classroom?
- Where do you see yourself in 10 years?
- What is the greatest obstacle you have had to overcome?
- What issues confront medicine today? (see www.healthpolitics.com)
- What has been your greatest achievement?
- What person, past or present, would you most like to meet?
- What have you read recently in the press about health care?
- What makes you a better applicant than others?
- Why do you want to become a physician?
- How would you express your concern for a child needing an amputation?
- How do you relax?
- What is your biggest concern about entering medical school?
- Describe your best teacher and what made her or him unique.
- Describe an experience you had helping others.
- What was the last book you read?
- Describe an experience where you were misjudged.

- What has been your favorite non-science course and why?
- Who are your senators, congressional representatives, governor?
- What was your most difficult or demoralizing experience?
- What is the difference between sympathy and empathy?
- Is there anything you want to brag about or that you need to explain?
- If you are accepted to multiple schools, how will you make your decision?
- What is the toughest thing about being a patient?
- What type of criticism upsets you?
- Have you ever been a patient and, if so, can you reveal how that felt?
- How have your personal and volunteer experiences strengthened your goal to become a physician?
- What have been the strengths and weaknesses of your college preparation?
- Would you say you are most like your father or mother, and why?
- Why did you choose an osteopathic/allopathic school?
- What will you do next year if you don't get into medical school?
- Is this school your first choice?
- Why did you apply to this medical school?
- Is there anything I haven't asked you that you want to tell me?

The following subjects were covered in over two-thirds of the Class of 2006's medical school interviews:

- The source of your inspiration to pursue medicine
- Interpersonal qualities that will enhance your practice of medicine
- Specific qualities that lead to choice of this medical school
- Qualities that will insure your success as a medical school student and physician
- Interest in generalist versus specialist fields

The following topics are commonly raised regarding medical ethics:

- Privacy
- Children's rights
- Rights of the handicapped
- Rights of the terminally ill
- Rights of defective newborns
- Organ donation
- Care of the mentally handicapped
- Care of the elderly
- Determination of death
- Physician's responsibility for societal health

3. Physical Appearance

Physical appearance creates a first impression and impacts how you are perceived. Present yourself in a personable and professional manner. Some dress for success tips:

- Dress conservatively. Men should wear a suit or a blazer and neatly pressed pants with a dress shirt and simple tie. Women should wear a suit or solid dress.

- Women should avoid distracting or flashy jewelry.
- Jackets should be free of lapel pins.
- Remove bulky items from pockets.
- Collar and tie should be straight. Scarves should be in place.
- Avoid half-glasses or light-sensitive ones that conceal your eyes.

4. Body Language

Physicians are expected to be skilled communicators whose facial expressions and hand gestures carry their message. Your body language is closely observed by a physician interviewer. The following gestures convey sincerity and interest:

- Make eye contact while you are listening.
- Sit erect but not stiff, leaning slightly forward.
- Use normal conversational hand movements to underscore your message.
- Listen intently to all questions and responses from the interviewer.

Avoid the following:

- Fidgeting or nervous gestures
- Inappropriate smiling or laughter
- Tightly grasping the arms of a chair or your hands in a prayer gesture
- Tightening and loosening your facial muscles
- Unnaturally straight, rigid posture
- Wandering eyes, particularly when you are addressed or speaking

Interview Recommendations

1. There is no consistency from one interviewer to the next. Styles and approaches vary. Expect anything.

2. Most interviews are open and non-combative. Approach the interview with optimism.

3. Honesty is key.

4. Be prepared for questions regarding weaknesses or discrepancies in your application.

5. Don't list any honors, research projects, or volunteer experiences in your application that you will be unable to support as real and significant.

6. Ask questions if you have real ones about the school.

7. Read the school catalogue prior to the interview.

8. Do not ask what your chances are.

9. Do not get upset if the interviewer is late.

10. Allow the interviewer to interrupt you, but don't interrupt the interviewer.

11. Elaborate, but don't dominate conversation.

12. Know your application file better than the interviewer (excluding your letters of recommendation).

13. Don't ask questions about your letters of recommendation if you have waived your right to see them.

14. Know something about the city you are visiting, even if only from that day's local newspaper or the taxi driver.

15. Don't try to second-guess the interviewer.

16. Avoid slang terms.

17. Be courteous and considerate toward all office staff.

18. If you know a student or faculty member personally, feel free to weave this naturally into the conversation, identifying her or him as a source of guidance and advice.

19. If this school is your first choice, state it. If not, explain your first choice if asked, and present this school as your second, if this is accurate.

20. If your choice of this school is tied to a fiancee's or spouse's choice, state it. Most schools are sympathetic to couples.

Optimal Arrival for the Interview

A thoroughly planned arrival tips the odds in your favor. If the interview is not in your immediate area, come the day before and stay overnight in a hotel or at a friend's home. Be sure that the accommodations are adequate for a good night's sleep and grooming the following morning. If possible, preview the physical site where the interview will take place. If you have the interview room number, arrive early to familiarize yourself with the location. Seeing the site with its physical arrangement avoids any sense of surprise that might shake your confidence during the interview. Awaken that morning with plenty of extra time so that you can properly groom, eat, and arrive with time to spare. Use the bathroom prior to the interview to check your clothes and your smile in the mirror.

Review the following quick tips for success:

1. Be honest

2. Be professional

3. Think fast, but speak slowly

4. Be human and interesting

5. Smile. Believe in yourself and you will transfer this belief to your interviewer.

Relaxation Techniques

Most candidates experience appropriate anxiety as they approach their interview. Remember that confidence is earned and you only acquire it by meeting challenges in a positive, determined spirit. If nervous in the final hour, try the following:

- Walk around the block, let your muscles relax, your eyes wander and b-r-e-a-t-h-e. Whistle. Sing.

- Stretch your arms, legs, torso and facial muscles.

- Think of treasured or humorous memories. Smile or laugh.

- Breathe deeply, counting for a number of seconds, then hold your breath the equivalent number of seconds and finally exhale for as long as you can. Repeat this, each time lengthening the breath, the hold and the exhalation.

- If you are in a room awaiting the interviewer's arrival, practice deep breathing and alternately tense and relax your muscles, head to toe.

- Acknowledge that even seasoned professionals experience some stage fright. If controlled, this energizes and enhances your performance.

- Remember to believe in the very best within you.

The Appearance

The interview begins when the interviewer enters the room. Rise and greet the interviewer professionally with a firm handshake and a smile. Express your pleasure and gratitude for the opportunity to interview at this medical school. While the interviewer will take the lead and ask the questions, it's important to keep in mind that you mutually own this interview. Ideally, you will enjoy an interpersonal exchange that connects and enriches you both.

Some key points:

1. Be personal and professional
Doctors may begin somewhat formally. Interviews often begin tensely and gradually yield to a warmer, more relaxed atmosphere. Mirror the mood of the interviewer and stay positive.

2. Stay on message
You should have in mind two or three points that you wish to convey during the interview. Seek opportunities early to introduce and reinforce these points.

3. Practice active listening
Listen carefully to questions posed. Clarify any inquiry or information that is unclear before you respond.

4. Control the pace
When nervous, most people speak too quickly. A controlled, slower pace shows a contemplative, more self-possessed candidate.

5. Monitor your body language
Be aware that your body is a powerful communication tool.

6. Stay alert, polite, poised

Skilled interviewers will attempt to relax you so that you will be honest and spontaneous with them. Their goal is to get to know the real you. This is your goal as well. Remember, though, that you need to maintain a polished, professional demeanor.

7. Maintain respectful, interested eye contact

Use eye contact as you would when fully engaged in an interesting conversation with a friend.

8. Affirm the positive

If asked a question that provides an opportunity to voice something you think is important, restate the question during your response. You might even reveal that you are glad the interviewer broached the subject.

9. Proceed mindfully

Stay within the bounds of a professional interview. The interviewer is not a trusted confidante or close friend. Rather, the interviewer is appraising your personal qualities and communication skills. Humor can jeopardize your candidacy. You needn't be stiff or refrain from smiling. Just save your favorite joke for a more appropriate audience.

10. Enjoy the interview and learn from it

At the end of your meeting, you will know more about the interviewer, yourself, and this prospective medical school. Your performance will be improved by an attitude that emphasizes exploration rather than fear.

Tough Questions...

Foresee tough questions or those that come from left field. Try to provide a reasonable and informed response. It is not so much what you say, but how you say it. Some counsel:

1. Acknowledge that this is a difficult question. This shows that you are listening and gives you a few moments to prepare a reasoned, balanced response.

2. Demonstrate concern and thoughtfulness in your response and maintain a moderate voice.

3. Above all, don't take a tough question personally. Often, an interviewer poses difficult questions to test your resilience.

4. Do not argue or become defensive. The last thing you want to do is dispute the interviewer.

5. Modulate your body language. You may want to verbally retaliate, but your body should do just the opposite. This softens the impact of the trying question and demonstrates your equilibrium.

6. Segue to a more favorable message. While addressing the question, relate it to a subject that contains some of the major messages you want to convey. Candidates who can turn the tables diplomatically prove their mettle and grace.

7. Don't be overwhelmed. Your whole life is not on the line. If one hard question can undo you, you may not be able to withstand the rigors of this demanding profession.

8. Conclude your response on an amicable, positive note.

Post Interview Self-Evaluation

Now that you have made it through the interview, your work isn't over. Breathe, walk, eat, and then sit down within an hour of your interview and answer the following questions:

1. Did I stay on message?

2. Was I in control?

3. Did I tell the truth and avoid exaggeration?

4. Was I calm and did I pace myself well?

5. Did I anticipate the questions?

6. Did I present a positive, professional image?

7. Did I listen carefully?

8. Was I a credible candidate?

9. Could I have done better and how?

10. What did I learn?

There's always something you could have done a little bit better. Through conscientious introspection, you will continually develop your interpersonal skills.

Summary of Interview Advice

In summation:

1. Be Prepared: Have something to say. Say it with style, force and intelligence.

2. Be Human: Medicine requires excellent communication and people skills, composure and poise. During your interview, demonstrate your maturity, thoughtfulness and sensitivity.

3. Be Yourself: Physicians regularly practice reading people's overt and covert responses. Be yourself, trust in your preparation and in human nature and learn from your experience.

Good luck!

V
The Profile

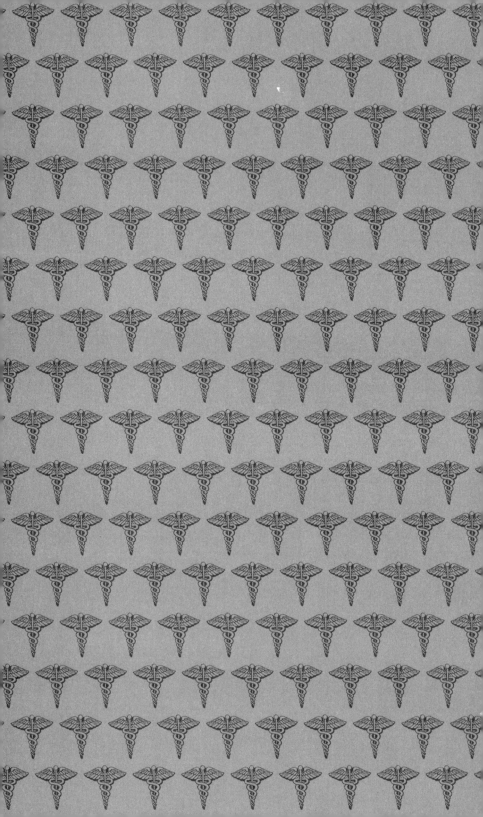

V   The Profile

Allopathic: Class of 2007

- 125 schools
- 34,786 applicants
- 17,539 entrants
- 50.4% acceptance
- 50.8% women
- 12.9% Black and Hispanic entrants

Average Admission Scores

MCAT
VR	9
PS	10
BS	10

GPA
Sciences	3.54
Total	3.61

Osteopathic: Class of 2007

- 20 schools
- 7,140 applicants
- 3,079 entrants
- 42% acceptance
- 47.5% women
- 8.6% Black and Hispanic entrants

Average Entrant Scores

MCAT
VR	8.06
PS	7.97
BS	8.5

GPA
Sciences	3.36
Total	3.43

Medical Students' Beliefs:

A 2003 survey of matriculating medical students conducted by the Association of American Medical Colleges revealed the following beliefs:

1. Physicians' legal liabilities and the high cost of malpractice insurance are major problems.
2. Physicians have an opportunity to exercise greater influence on health promotion and disease.
3. Everyone is entitled to receive adequate medical care regardless of his ability to pay.
4. Changes in the healthcare system are impairing physician's independence.
5. Advances in the biomedical sciences and their application to the care of patients will make the practice of medicine more challenging and rewarding in the near future.
6. Access to medical care continues to be a major problem in the United States.
7. Animal research is necessary for the advancement of medicine.
8. Having interesting and intelligent colleagues is a major benefit of being a physician.
9. Physicians have an obligation to care for a reasonable number of patients who will be unable to pay for the services they receive.
10. Care of the chronically ill is one of the most challenging aspects of being a doctor.

Top five reasons for choosing medicine:

1. Opportunity to make a difference.

2. Educate patients about health.

3. Exercise social responsibility.

4. Contact with patients.

5. Intellectual challenge and critical thinking.

Top five reasons students chose a particular medical school:

1. Friendliness of administrators, faculty, and students.

2. Geographic location.

3. Teaching methods of school.

4. School's ability to place students in residency programs.

5. General reputation of school.

CLASS OF 2007

Medical School	Class Size	% In-State Pupils	% Women	Resident Tuition	Non-Resident Tuition
Alabama					
University of Alabama*	160	90	37	8,886	26,658
University of South Alabama*	64	92	59	9,770	16,400
Arizona					
Arizona College of Medicine§	140	27	44	32,251	32,251
University of Arizona	110	98	53	11,483	N/A
Arkansas					
University of Arkansas	147	98	53	11,642	23,284
California					
University of California Davis*	96	100	50	0	12,245
University of California Irvine*	92	99	46	0	12,245
University of California Los Angeles*	121	88	50	0	12,245
University of California San Diego*	121	92	54	0	12,245
University of California San Francisco*	141	82	58	0	12,245
Loma Linda University	165	48	52	30,012	30,012
University of Southern California	160	81	47	35,928	35,928
Stanford University	87	47	50	34,716	34,716
Touro University College of Osteopathic Medicine§	131	60	48.7	29,650	29,650
Western University of the Health Sciences*§	174	66	51	31,115	31,115
Colorado					
University of Colorado	130	80	45	15,333	67,000
Connecticut					
University of Connecticut*	74	72	66	12,000	27,300
Yale University	100	22	54	33,800	33,800

CLASS OF 2007

Medical School	Class Size	% In-State Pupils	% Women	Resident Tuition	Non-Resident Tuition
Washington, DC					
George Washington University	167	1	56	39,005	39,005
Georgetown University	170	0	52	33,670	33,670
Howard University	111	3	56	20,010	20,010
Florida					
Nova Southeastern University§	207	54.7	52	22,265	27,955
Florida State	46	100	41	14,208	43,530
University of Florida	85	100	55	13,925	40,082
University of Miami	141	75	46	28,050	36,740
University of South Florida*	115	100	46	13,925	41,782
Georgia					
Emory University	113	32	52	32,576	32,576
Medical College of Georgia	180	98	43	9,772	29,976
Mercer University	60	100	47	26,372	26,372
Morehouse School of Medicine*	52	52	67	20,966	20,966
Hawaii					
University of Hawaii	62	90	66	14,808	28,512
Illinois					
Chicago College of OM	185	25	47	36,740	36,740
University of Chicago Pritzker	104	39	52	29,046	29,046
Rosalind Franklin University of Medicine and Science/ Chicago Medical School	184	25	47	36,740	36,740
University of Illinois	313	81	41	20,874	48,310
Loyola University of Chicago	140	42	50	32,800	32,800
Northwestern University	170	27	50	34,998	34,998
Rush Medical College	120	79	56.6	32,268	32,268
Southern Illinois University	72	100	54	16,149	48,447
Indiana					
Indiana University	280	95	72	17,993	36,827

CLASS OF 2007

Medical School	Class Size	% In-State Pupils	% Women	Resident Tuition	Non-Resident Tuition
Iowa					
University of Iowa	142	68	50	17,838	36,306
Des Moines University of Osteopathic Medicine and Surgery§ *	201	25	44	29,050	29,050
Kansas					
University of Kansas	175	87	42	14,584	29,115
Kentucky					
University of Kentucky	95	92	44	13,604	31,996
University of Louisville	149	82	46	14,544	36,262
Pikeville College School of Osteopathic Medicine (PCSOM)§	73	45	47	27,000	27,000
Louisiana					
Louisiana State–New Orleans*	167	99	50	10,426	24,574
Louisiana State–Shreveport	100	100	40	8,846	22,994
Tulane University	155	25	42	34,986	34,986
Maine					
University of New England COM§	121	14.5	51	30,990	30,990
Maryland					
Johns Hopkins University*	119	15	53	30,900	30,900
University of Maryland*	150	75	61	17,493	32,558
Uniformed Service University	167	N/A	40	0	0
Massachusetts					
Boston University	155	15	49.67	36,530	36,530
Harvard Medical School	165	8	51	32,000	32,000
University of Massachusetts*	100	100	57	8,352	N/A
Tufts University	170	29	43	39,579	39,579

CLASS OF 2007

Medical School	Class Size	% In-State Pupils	% Women	Resident Tuition	Non-Resident Tuition
Michigan					
College of Osteopathic Medicine§	143	92	53	20,750	44,450
Michigan State University	106	80	54	19,726	43,256
University of Michigan	170	45	43	19,708	30,708
Wayne State University	257	88	46	16,873.20	35,114
Minnesota					
Mayo Medical School	44	25	45	11,250	22,500
University of Minnesota –Duluth	54	86	40	25,073	46,581
University of Minnesota –Minneapolis	165	127	50	25,073	46,581
Mississippi					
University of Mississippi	101	100	41	6,938	13,298
Missouri					
Kirksville COM§	168	22	41	31,700	31,700
Kansas City University of Medicine and Biosciences§	232	12	46	31,200	31,200
University of Missouri –Columbia	96	96	43	18,792	34,418
University of Missouri –Kansas City	124	82	49	25,094	50,405
St. Louis University	158	29	44	36,190	36,190
Washington University	122	12	46	37,032	37,032
Nebraska					
Creighton University	120	12	48	35,364	35,364
University of Nebraska	118	88	40	16,640	39,020

CLASS OF 2007

Medical School	Class Size	% In-State Pupils	% Women	Resident Tuition	Non-Resident Tuition
Nevada					
University of Nevada	52	90	50	9,232	26,810
New Hampshire					
Dartmouth Medical School	78	15	55	31,600	31,600
New Jersey					
University of Medicine and Dentristy of NJ	170	84*	51	19,776	30,947
*all out-of-state students qualified for in-state tuition					
UMDNJ –Robert Wood Johnson	156	88	54	19,776	30,947
UMDNJ–School of OM§	96	97	52	19,776	30,947
New Mexico					
University of New Mexico	75	96	58.7	10,369	29,805
New York					
Albany Medical College	133	34	51	38,860	38,860
Albert Einstein COM	180	47	59	34,375	34,375
Columbia University*	150	33	50	35,036	35,036
Cornell University Weill Medical College	101	38	54	30,170	30,170
Mt.Sinai SOM	120	38	58	31,250	31,250
New York COM§	305	64	57	28,863	28,863
New York Medical College	187	34	50	34,040	34,040
New York University*	160	43	51	26,750	26,750
University of Rochester*	100	42	54	31,500	31,500
State University of NY –Downstate	180	89	49	16,800	29,900
University of Buffalo	135	86	56	16,800	29,900
State University of NY –Stony Brook	101	98	52	16,800	29,900
State University of NY –Upstate (Syracuse)	151	86	42	16,800	29,900

CLASS OF 2007

Medical School	Class Size	% In-State Pupils	% Women	Resident Tuition	Non-Resident Tuition
North Carolina					
Duke University*	100	9	51	29,706	31,194
The Brody School of Medicine at East Carolina University	72	100	37	3,602	28,524
University of NC Chapel Hill	160	89	52	7,385	33,524
Wake Forrest University SOM	108	37	44	32,056	32,056
North Dakota					
University of North Dakota	61	77	54	15,343	40,963
Ohio					
Case Western Reserve	146	50	50	36,500	36,500
University of Cincinnati	158	75	41	18,630	33,159
Medical College of Ohio	156	75	39	16,800	36,500
Northeastern Ohio University	37	89	46	18,255	36,510
Ohio State University	210	62	39	18,927	36,510
Ohio University COM§	107	85	56	18,015	26,253
Wright State University	95	88	53	16,602	23,496
Oklahoma					
Oklahoma State University COM§	88	99	46	13,774	30,144
University of Oklahoma	142	95	55	13,234	33,611
Oregon					
Oregon Health Sciences*	107	51	63	21,000	31,500
Pennsylvania					
Lake Erie COM§	214	38	46	24,100	25,100
Jefferson Medical College	229	45	51	34,565	34,565
Drexel University COM	250	28	46	33,1000	33,100
Pennsylvania State University	125	41	57	26,062	36,232
Philadelphia COM§	264	54.7	59.8	30,576	30,576
University of Pennsylvania	147	31	43	34,482	34,482
University of Pittsburgh	145	36	48	30,084	35,876
Temple University	177	60	46	30,020	36,760

CLASS OF 2007

Medical School	Class Size	% In-State Pupils	% Women	Resident Tuition	Non-Resident Tuition
Puerto Rico					
Universidad Central del Caribe*	62	82	NOT AVAILABLE	18,000	25,000
Ponce School of Medicine	66	68	45	17,836	26,590
University of Puerto Rico	115	100	49	5,000	10,000
Rhode Island					
Brown University	69	17	53	31,872	31,872
South Carolina					
Medical University of South Carolina*	144	95	45	4,544	14,604
University of South Carolina	83	88	45	16,900	48,870
South Dakota					
University of South Dakota*	50	88	46	12,498	29,937
Tennessee					
East Tennessee State University	60	95	45	15,110	30,800
Meharry Medical College*	80	20	45	26,352	26,352
University of Tennessee	150	95	42	16,048	31,962
Vanderbilt University	104	15	39	30,100	30,100
Texas					
Baylor College of Medicine*	168	49	45	15,110	15,110
Texas A&M	74	93	59	6,550	19,650
Texas College of OM§	127	96.1	58	6,550	19,650
Texas Tech University	130	95	41	7,654	20,754
University of Texas–Dallas	218	89	40	7,660	20,760
University of Texas –Galveston*	205	94	41	7,450	20,550
University of Texas –Houston	202	96	47	8,275	21,375
University of Texas –San Antonio*	204	96	42	6,550	19,650

CLASS OF 2007

Medical School	Class Size	% In-State Pupils	% Women	Resident Tuition	Non-Resident Tuition
Utah					
University of Utah	102	75	32	13,297	25,172
Vermont					
University of Vermont	100	28	50	22,300	39,020
Virginia					
Eastern Virginia Medical School	110	55	44	18,975	35,075
Edward Via Virginia College of OM§	154	28.6	47.9	28,300	28,300
Virginia Commonwealth University	184	54	47	18,500	34,328
University of Virginia	140	66	50	21,500	33,000
Washington					
University of Washington	178	93	48	12,448	29,388
West Virginia					
Marshall University	53	87	49	12,190	32,020
West Virginia School of OM§	103	49	48	15,272	37,794
West Virginia University SOM	108	74	40	12,366	30,106
Wisconsin					
Medical College of Wisconsin	205	48	46	26,094	31,150
University of Wisconsin	150	87	54	21,153	32,277

* The tuition figures above do not include student fees. Student fees range from $500 to $1,500 for most schools. Schools marked with an asterisk have student fees ranging from $2,500 to $7,000.

Contact schools directly to confirm current student tuition and fees.

§ Denotes osteopathic medical school.

N/A   Denotes not applicable.

VI
Informational Resources

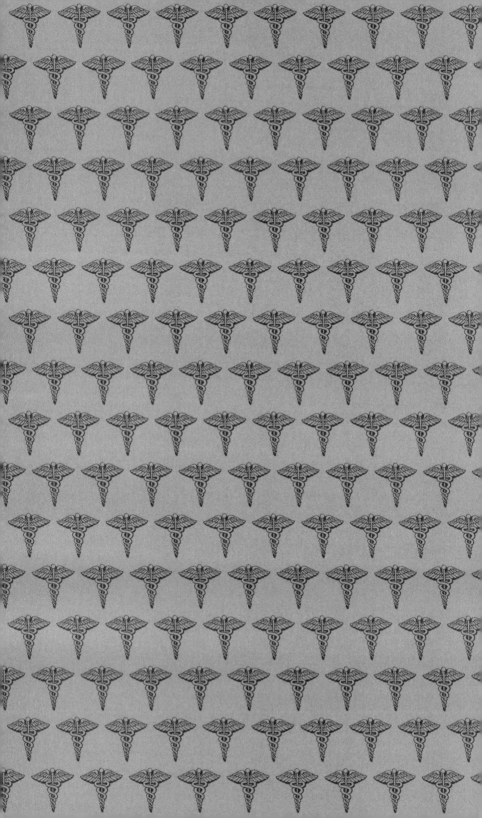

VI Informational Resources

Print Information

These printed resources may be useful supplements to your educational and financial planning:

1. *The Student Guide, 2004-2005.* Department of Education. Free. EDPubs. P.O. Box 1398, Jessup, M.D. 20794-1398 (877) 433-7827; www.edpubs.org

2. *The College Board Book of Major , 2005.* Item #007018. $24.95, plus sales tax where applicable. Revised annually. College Board Publications, P.O. Box 869010, Plano, TX 75074; 800-323-7155; www.collegeboard.com

3. *Need a Lift? College Financial Aid Handbook, 2005.* Item #75207.5. $3.00 prepaid, plus sales tax where applicable and shipping and handling. The American Legion Emblem Sales, P.O. Box 1050, Indianapolis, IN 46206; (888) 453-4466

4. *Medical School Admission Requirements United States and Canada 2005-2006.* $25.00 plus shipping. Association of American Medical Colleges, 2450 N Street, NW, Washington, DC 20037; (202) 828-0416; www.aamc.org

5. *Health Professions Career & Education Directory, 2004-2005 edition.* $65.00, non-members; $55.00 members, plus shipping and handling. Order No. OP-417504BXY. American Medical Association, P.O. Box 930876, Atlanta, GA 31193-0876; Attn: Order Department; Email meded@ama-assn.org for an order form, or call (800) 621-8335 to have one faxed to you.

6. *300 Ways To Put Your Talent To Work in the Health Field.* $18.00, non-members; $15.00, members, plus $5.00 shipping and handling. National Health Council, 1730 M Street, NW, Suite 500, Washington, DC 20036; (202) 785-3910; go to www.nationalhealthcouncil.org to order.

7. *Essays That Will Get You into Medical School.* By Dan Kaufman, Chris Dowhan, $12.95 paperback, Barrons Educational Series, Inc., 250 Wireless Blvd, Hauppauge NY, 11788; 1-800-645-3476

8. *The Pact.* By Rameck Hunt, Samson Davis, Lisa Page, George Jenkins,. $14.00 paperback, Riverhead Books, Penguin Group (USA) Inc., 405 Murray Hill Parkway, East Rutherford, NJ 07073; 1-800-788-6262

Health Careers Information

These professional associations provide information useful to health professionals:

1. Association of American Medical Colleges
    2450 N Street, NW
    Washington, DC 20037
    (202) 828-0400
    web site: www.aamc.org

2. American Association of Colleges of Osteopathic Medicine
    Suite 310
    5550 Friendship Boulevard
    Chevy Chase, MD 20815-7231
    (301) 968-4100
    web site: www.aacom.org

3. American Association of Colleges of Pharmacy
    1426 Prince Street
    Alexandria, VA 22314-2841
    (703) 739-2330
    web site: www.aacp.org

4. American Association of Colleges of Podiatric Medicine
    Suite 320
    1580 Crabbs Branch Way
    Rockville, MD 20850-4307
    (800) 443-3514
    web site: www.aacpm.org

5. American Dental Education Association
    Suite 1100
    1400 K Street, NW
    Washington, DC 20005
    (202) 289-7201
    web site: www.adea.org

6. Association of American Veterinary Medical Colleges
    Suite 301
    1101 Vermont Avenue, NW
    Washington, DC 20005-3521
    (202) 371-9195
    web site: www.aavmc.org

7. Association of Schools and Colleges of Optometry
    Suite 510
    6110 Executive Boulevard
    Rockville, MD 20852
    (301) 231-5944
    web site: www.opted.org

8. Association of Schools of Public Health
    1101 15th Street, NW
    Suite 910
    Washington, DC 20005
    (202) 296-1099
    web site: www.asph.org

9. National Association of Advisors to the Health Professions
    P.O. Box 1518
    Champaign, IL 61824
    (217) 355-0063
    web site: www.naahp.org

10. Alpha Epsilon Delta
    National Office
    James Madison University
    MSC 4307
    Harrisonburg, VA 22807
    (540) 568-2594
    web site: www.jmu.edu/orgs/nationalaed

Electronic Information:

www.positiveprofiles.com – Pfizer Medical Humanities Initiative; offers email access to medical schools nationwide, publications, scholarship information, physician profiles, inspirational stories, links to other resources.

www.aamc.org – offers information on America's 125 allopathic medical schools.

www.aamc.org/students/financing/md2/start.htm – (MD)2 : Monetary Decisions for Medical Doctors is a comprehensive, three-part program developed by the AAMC to assist premedical and medical students in their planning for the financial aspects of their medical education.

http://services.aamc.org/postbac/ – AAMC's database of post-baccalaurate premedical programs.

www.aacom.org – offers information on America's 20 osteopathic medical schools.

www.ama-assn.org/go/becominganmd – offers information on becoming an M.D.

www.ama-assn.org/ama/pub/category/2322.html – offers information on careers in allied health professions.

www.kaplan.com – offers MCAT preparation and information.

www.healthpolitics.com – a weekly, Internet-based electronic media program that explores complex topics at the intersection of health-care and policy.

www.review.com – offers MCAT preparation and information.

www.naahp.org – National Association of Advisors for the Health Professions

www.asph.org – Association of Schools of Public Health

www.jmu.edu/orgs/nationalaed – national medical honor society, Alpha Epsilon Delta

www.aacp.org – American Association of Colleges of Pharmacy

www.aacpm.org – American Association of Colleges of Podiatric Medicine

www.adea.org – American Dental Education Association

www.aavmc.org – Association of American Veterinary Medical Colleges

www.opted.org – Association of Schools and Colleges of Optometry

Medical Science Information:

www.ama-assn.org – The American Medical Association

www.cmwf.org – The Commonwealth Fund

www.drkoop.com – Dr. Koop

www.jama.ama-assn.org – The Journal of the American Medical Association

www.mayohealth.org – Mayo Clinic Health Oasis

www.nhionline.net – National Health Information

www.nih.gov – National Institutes of Health

www.nejm.org – The New England Journal of Medicine

www.pfizer.com – Pfizer Inc

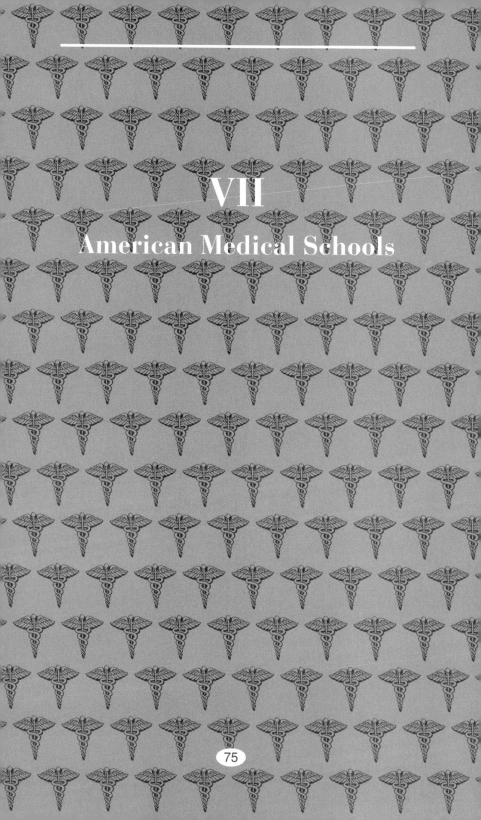

VII
American Medical Schools

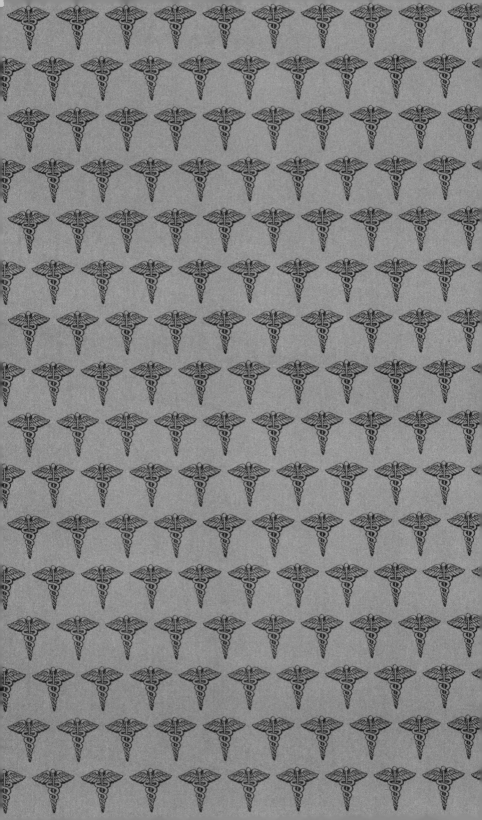

VII American Medical Schools

Admissions Contact Person & Address

ALABAMA

University of Alabama
  School of Medicine
Dr. Nathan Smith
Assistant Dean for Admissions
Office of Medical Student
  Services/Admissions VH-100
Birmingham, AL 35294-0019
205-934-2333

University of South Alabama
  College of Medicine
Mark Scott
Director for Admissions
Office of Admissions 241 CSAB
Mobile, AL 36688-0002
251-460-7176

ARIZONA

Arizona College of Osteopathic
  Medicine[§]
Jim Walter
Director of Admissions
19555 N. 59th Avenue
Glendale, AZ 85308
888-247-9277

University of Arizona
  College of Medicine
Dr. Christopher Leadem
Senior Associate Dean for
  Admissions and Student Affairs
Admissions Office
P.O. Box 245075
Tucson, AZ 85724-5075
520-626-6214

ARKANSAS

University of Arkansas for Medical
  Sciences College of Medicine
Tom G. South
Director of Student Admissions
  and Financial Aid
4301 W. Markham St., Slot 551
Little Rock, AK 72205-7199
501-686-5354

CALIFORNIA

University of California–
  Davis School of Medicine
Dr. Edward Dagang
Associate Dean for Student Affairs
Admissions Office
1 Shield Avenue
Davis, CA 95616
530-752-2717

University of California–
  Irvine College of Medicine
Gayle Pierce
Director of Admissions
P.O. Box 4089
Medical Education Bldg., 802
Irvine, CA 92697-5981
949-824-5388

University of California–
  Los Angeles
  UCLA School of Medicine
Dr. Neil Parker
Senior Associate Dean for
  Admissions
P.O. Box 951720
Office of Student Affairs
159 Center for Health Sciences
Los Angeles, CA 90095-1720
310-825-6081

University of California–
   San Diego
   School of Medicine
Dr. David Rapaport
Acting Associate Dean for
   Admissions
UCSDSOM Admission
0621/Medical Teaching Facility
9500 Gilman Drive
LaJolla, CA 92093-0621
858-534-3880

University of California–
   San Francisco
   School of Medicine
Dr. Henry Ralston
Associate Dean of Admissions
521 Parnass Avenue
C-200, Box 0408
San Francisco, CA 94143-0408
415-476-4044

Loma Linda University
   School of Medicine
Stephen Nyirady, Ph.D.
Associate Dean for Admissions
11234 Anderson Street, MC A-500
Loma Linda, CA 92350
909-558-4467

University of Southern California
   School of Medicine
Dr. Erin Quinn
Dean of Admissions
1975 Zonal Avenue (KAM 100-C)
Los Angeles, CA 90089-9021
323-442-2552

Stanford University
   School of Medicine
Dr. Gabriel Garcia
Associate Dean for Medical School
   Admissions
251 Campus Drive
MSOB Room X335
Stanford, CA 94305-5404
650-724-5516

Touro University
   College of Osteopathic Medicine[§]
Dr. Donald Haight
Director of Admissions
1310 Johnson Lane
Vallejo, CA 94592
888-887-7336

Western University of the Health
   Sciences/College of Osteopathic
   Medicine of the Pacific[§]
Susan Hanson
Director of Admissions
309 East 2nd Street
Pomona, CA 91766-1854
909-469-5335

COLORADO

University of Colorado
   School of Medicine
Dr. Henry Sondheimer
Associate Dean for Admissions
4200 E. Ninth Avenue, C-297
Denver, CO 80262
303-315-7361

CONNECTICUT

University of Connecticut
   School of Medicine
Keat Sanford, Ph.D.
Assistant Dean
263 Farmington Ave., Rm AG-062
Farmington, CT 06030-3906
860-679-4306

Yale University
   School of Medicine
Dr. Thomas L. Lentz
Associate Dean – Admissions
Office of Admissions
367 Cedar Street
New Haven, CT 06510
203-785-2643

WASHINGTON, DC

George Washington University
   School of Medicine and Health
   Sciences
Dianne McQuail
Dean for Admissions
Ross Hall 716
2300 Eye Street, NW, Room 716
Washington, DC 20037
202-994-3506

Georgetown University
   School of Medicine
Eugene T. Ford
Director of Admissions
Office of Admissions
3900 Reservoir Road, NW
Washington, DC 20007
202-687-1154

Howard University
   College of Medicine
Ann Finney
Admissions Officer
520 W Street, NW
Washington, DC 20059
202-806-6270

FLORIDA

Nova Southeastern University
   College of Osteopathic Medicine§
Marla Frohlinger
Vice Chancellor – Student Affairs
3200 S. University Drive
Fort Lauderdale, FL 33328
954-262-1101

Florida State University
   College of Medicine
Dr. Helen Livingston
Assistant Dean for Student Affairs
   and Admissions
Administration Building, Room 117
Tallahassee, FL 32306-4300
850-644-7904

University of Florida
   College of Medicine
Dr. Ira Gessner
Chair, Medical Selection Committee
P.O. Box 100216
J. Hillis Miller Health Center
Gainesville, FL 32610
352-392-4569

University of Miami
   School of Medicine
Dr. R.E. Hinkley
Associate Dean for Admissions
P.O. Box 016159
Miami, FL 33101
305-243-6791

University of South Florida
   College of Medicine
Dr. Steve Specter
Associate Dean of Admissions and
   Student Affairs
P.O. Box 3
12901 Bruce B. Downs Blvd.
MDC3
Tampa, FL 33612-4799
813-974-2229

GEORGIA

Emory University
   School of Medicine
Dr. J. William Eley
Associate Dean/Director of
   Admissions
Woodruff Health Sciences Building
1440 Clifton Road, NE, Room 115
Atlanta, GA 30322
404-727-5660

Medical College of Georgia
   School of Medicine
Dr. Mason Thompson
Associate Dean for Admissions
AA-2040
Augusta, GA 30912-4760
706-721-3186

Mercer University
School of Medicine
Dr. A. Peter Eveland
Associate Dean for Admissions
Office of Admissions & Student
Affairs
1550 College Street
Macon, GA 31207-0001
478-301-2542

Morehouse School of Medicine
Dr. Angela Franklin
Associate Dean – Student Affairs/
Admissions
720 Westview Drive, SW
Atlanta, GA 30310-1495
404-752-1650

HAWAII

University of Hawaii
John A. Burns School of Medicine
Dr. Satoru Izutsu
Senior Associate Dean/Chair, Adm
Com
1960 East-West Road
Honolulu, HI 96822
808-956-5505

ILLINOIS

Chicago College of Osteopathic
Medicine[§]
Mark Clancy
Director of Admissions
555 31st Street
Downer's Grove, IL 60515
630-515-7200

University of Chicago
Pritzker School of Medicine
Sylvia Robertson
Associate Dean of Admissions
924 E. 57th Street, BLSC 104
Chicago, IL 60637-5416
773-702-1937

Rosalind Franklin University
of Medicine and Science
Chicago Medical School
Kristine A. Jones
Director of Admissions
3333 Green Bay Road
N. Chicago, IL 60064
847-578-3206

University of Illinois
College of Medicine
Dr. Jorge A. Girotti
Associate Dean and Director of
Admissions
808 S. Wood Street
Room 165 CME M/C 783
Chicago, IL 60612-7302
312-996-5635

Loyola University Chicago
Stritch School of Medicine
LaDonna E. Norstrom
Assistant Dean, Admissions
Office of Admissions
2160 S. First Avenue
Building 120, Room 200
Maywood, IL 60153
708-216-3229

Northwestern University
Medical School
Dolores Brown
Associate Dean for Admissions
Morton 1-606
303 E. Chicago Avenue
Chicago, IL 60611-3008
312-503-8206

Rush Medical College of Rush
University
Jan L. Schmidt
Director of Admissions
524 Academic Facility
600 S. Paulina Street
Suite 524
Chicago, IL 60612
312-942-6913

Southern Illinois University
  School of Medicine
Erin L. Graham
Director of Admissions
Office of Student Affairs
P.O. Box 19624
Springfield, IL 62794-9624
217-545-6013

INDIANA

Indiana University
  School of Medicine
Mr. Robert M. Stump, Jr.
Director of Admissions
Fesler Hall 213
1120 South Drive
Indianapolis, IN 46202-5113
317-274-3772

IOWA

University of Iowa
  College of Medicine
Catherine Solow
Director of Admissions
100 Medicine Administration
  Building
Iowa City, IA 52242-1101
319-335-8052

Des Moines University
  College of Osteopathic Medicine§
Becky Grissom
Director of Admissions &
  Enrollment Development
3200 Grand Avenue
Des Moines, IA 50312
515-271-1499

KANSAS

University of Kansas
  School of Medicine
Sandra J. McCurdy, M.Ed.
Assistant Dean for Admissions
3901 Rainbow Boulevard
Kansas City, KS 66160-7301
913-588-5280

KENTUCKY

University of Kentucky
  College of Medicine
Dr. Carol L. Elam
Assistant Dean for Admissions
Admissions Room MN-102
Office of Student Affairs
800 Rose Street
Lexington, KY 40536-0298
859-323-6161

University of Louisville
  School of Medicine
Dr. Stephen F. Wheeler
Associate Dean of Admissions
Health Sciences Center
323 East Chestnut Street
Louisville, KY 40202-3866
502-852-5193

Pikeville College
  School of Osteopathic Medicine
  (PCSOM)§
Angel Hamilton
Director of Admissions
147 Sycamore Street
Pikeville, KY 41501-1194
606-218-5406

LOUISIANA

Louisiana State University
  Health Sciences Center,
  New Orleans
Dr. Sam G. McClugage
Associate Dean for Admissions
1901 Perdido Street, Box P3-4
New Orleans, LA 70112-1393
504-568-6262

Louisiana State University
  School of Medicine in Shreveport
Dr. F. Scott Kennedy
Assistant Dean for Student
  Admissions
P.O. Box 33932
1501 Kings Highway
Shreveport, LA 71130-3932
318-675-5190

Tulane University
  School of Medicine
Dr. Joseph C. Pisano
Associate Dean
1430 Tulane Avenue, SL67
New Orleans, LA 70112-2699
504-588-5187

MAINE

University of New England
  College Osteopathic Medicine[§]
Lisa Lane
Asst. Director Medical Admissions
11 Hills Beach Road
Biddeford, ME 04005
207-283-0171, ext. 2218

MARYLAND

Johns Hopkins University
  School of Medicine
Dr. James Weiss
Associate Dean for Admissions
733 North Broadway, Suite G-49
Baltimore, MD 21205-2196
410-955-3182

University of Maryland
  School of Medicine
Dr. Milford M. Foxwell, Jr.
Associate Dean for Admissions
Room 1-005, 655 W. Baltimore St.
Baltimore, MD 21201
410-706-7478

Uniformed Services University of
  the Health Sciences
Peter J. Stavish, L.T.C, M.S., U.S.A. (Ret)
Assistant Dean for Admissions &
  Academic Records
Admissions Office
4301 Jones Bridge Road
Bethesda, MD 20814-4799
301-295-3101

MASSACHUSETTS

Boston University
  School of Medicine
Dr. Robert Witzburg
Associate Dean for Admissions
Building L, Room 124
715 Albany Street
Boston, MA 02118
617-638-4630

Harvard Medical School
Robert J. Mayer, M.D.
Faculty Associate Dean for
  Admissions
25 Shattuck Street
Gordon Hall 210
Boston, MA 02115-6092
617-432-1550

University of Massachusetts
  Medical School
Dr. Jon Paraskos
Associate Dean for Admissions
55 Lake Avenue, N
Worcester, MA 01655
508-856-2323

Tufts University
  School of Medicine
Thomas M. Slavin
Director of Admissions
136 Harrison Avenue
Boston, MA 02111
617-636-6571

MICHIGAN

Michigan State University
  College of Osteopathic Medicine§
Kathie Schaefer
Director of Admissions
C110 East Fee Hall
East Lansing, MI 48824-1316
517-353-7740

Michigan State University
  College of Human Medicine
Christine L. Shafer, M.D.
Asst. Dean, Admissions
A-239 Life Sciences
East Lansing, MI 48824-1317
517-353-9620

University of Michigan
  Medical School
Dr. Daniel Remick
Dean, Admissions
D4303, Medical Science Building 1
1301 Catherine
Ann Arbor, MI 48109-0624
734-764-6317

Wayne State University
  School of Medicine
Dr. Silas Norman
Assistant Dean for Admissions
540 E. Canfield
Detroit, MI 48201
313-577-1466

MINNESOTA

Mayo Medical School
Dr. Patricia Barrier
Associate Dean for Student Affairs
200 First Street, SW
Rochester, MN 55905
507-284-3671

University of Minnesota
  Medical School
Duluth Campus
Dr. Lillian Repesh
Assoc. Dean for Admissions/
  Student Affairs, Duluth
Room 180
10 University Drive
Duluth, MN 55812
218-726-8511
Minneapolis Campus
Dr. Marilyn Becker
Director of Admissions, Twin Cities
MMC – 293
420 Delaware Street, SE
Minneapolis, MN 55455-0310
612-625-7977

MISSISSIPPI

University of Mississippi
  School of Medicine
Dr. Steven Case
Associate Dean – Admissions
2500 N. State Street
Jackson, MS 39216-4505
601-984-5010

MISSOURI

Kirksville College of Osteopathic
  Medicine§
Lori A. Haxton, M.A.
Assistant to Vice President for
  Admissions and Alumni Services
800 West Jefferson Street
Kirksville, MO 63501
866-626-2878 or 660-626-2237

Kansas City University of Medicine
  and Biosciences§
Leann Carlton
Executive Director of Student
  Services and Admissions
1750 Independence Avenue
Kansas City, MO 64106-1453
816-283-2350

University of Missouri–
  Columbia School of Medicine
Judy Nolke
Admissions Coordinator
MA213-215,
Medical Science Building
One Hospital Drive
Columbia, MO 65212
573-882-2923

University of Missouri–Kansas City*
  School of Medicine
Mary Anne Morgenegg
Admissions Coordinator
Counsel on Selection
2411 Holmes Street
Kansas City, MO 64108
816-235-1870

St. Louis University
  School of Medicine
Dr. James Willmore
Associate Dean of Admissions
1402 S. Grand Boulevard
St. Louis, MO 63104
314-977-9870

Washington University
School of Medicine
Dr. W. Edwin Dodson
Associate Dean for Admissions
660 S. Euclid Avenue, #8107
St. Louis, MO 63110
314-362-6858

NEBRASKA

Creighton University
  School of Medicine
Dr. Henry Nipper
Assistant Dean
Medical School Admissions
Office of Admissions
2500 California Plaza
Omaha, NE 68178
402-280-2799

University of Nebraska
  College of Medicine
Dr. Jeffrey W. Hill
Assoc. Dean of Admissions and
  Student Affairs
Office of Admissions
986585 Nebraska Medical Center
Omaha, NE 68198-6585
402-559-6140

NEVADA

University of Nevada
  School of Medicine
Cheryl Hug-English
Associate Dean of Admissions and
  Student Affairs
Office of Admissions and
  Student Affairs
Mail Stop 357
Reno, NV 89557
775-784-6063

NEW HAMPSHIRE

Dartmouth Medical School
Andrew G. Welch
Director of Admissions
3 Rope Ferry Road
Hanover, NH 03755-1404
603-650-1505

NEW JERSEY

University of Medicine and
 Dentistry of NJ
 New Jersey Medical School
Dr. George F. Heinrich
Associate Dean for Admissions
185 S. Orange Avenue
Newark, NJ 07103
973-972-4631

University of Medicine and
 Dentistry of NJ
 Robert Wood Johnson Medical
 School
Dr. David Seiden
Associate Dean for Admissions
Admissions Office
675 Hoes Lane
Piscataway, NJ 08854
732-235-4576

University of Medicine and
 Dentistry of New Jersey
 School of Osteopathic Medicine[§]
Warren Wallace, Ed.D.
Associate Dean of Academics and
 Student Affairs
Office of Admissions, Suite 210
2nd Floor Academic Center
One Medical Center Drive
Stratford, NJ 08084
856-566-7050

NEW MEXICO

University of New Mexico
 School of Medicine
Dr. Roger Radloff
Assistant Dean for Admissions
Office of Admissions
MSCO8 – 4690 #1
Albuquerque, NM 87131-0001
505-272-3814

NEW YORK

Albany Medical College
Joanne H. Nanos
Director of Admissions and
 Student Records
Office of Admissions, MC3
47 New Scotland Avenue
Albany, NY 12208
518-262-5521

Albert Einstein College of Medicine
 of Yeshiva University
Noreen Kerrigan
Assistant Dean for Student
 Admissions
Jack & Pearl Resnick Campus
1300 Morris Park Avenue
Bronx, NY 10461
718-430-2106

Columbia University
 College of Physicians and
 Surgeons
Dr. Andrew G. Frantz
Associate Dean for Admissions
Admissions Office, Room 1-416
P.O. Box 41
630 West 168th Street
New York, NY 10032
212-305-3595

Cornell University Weill Medical
College
Dr. Charles Bardes
Associate Dean/Chair, Admissions
Committee
Room 104
445 East 69th Street
New York, NY 10021
212-746-1067

Mt. Sinai School of Medicine
Dr. Scott Barnett
Dean for Admissions
Annenberg Building, Room 5-04
1 Gustave L. Levy Pl.
New York, NY 10029
212-241-6696

New York College of Osteopathic
Medicine of NY Institute of
Technology§
Michael J. Schaefer
Director of Admissions
P.O. Box 8000
Old Westbury, NY 11568
516-686-3700

New York Medical College
Dr. Fern Juster
Associate Dean/Chair, Admissions
Committee
Sunshine Cottage
Valhalla, NY 10595
914-594-4507

New York University
School of Medicine*
Raymond J. Brienza
Assistant Dean for Admissions
P.O. Box 1924
New York, NY 10016
212-263-5290

University of Rochester
School of Medicine and Dentistry
Pat Samuelson
Director of Admissions
Medical Center
601 Elmwood Avenue, Box 601-A
Rochester, NY 14642
585-275-4539

State University of New York –
Health Science Center at
Brooklyn College of Medicine
Thomas Sabia
Assistant Dean of Admissions
450 Clarkson Avenue, Box 60M
Brooklyn, NY 11203
718-270-2446

University of Buffalo
School of Medicine and
Biomedical Sciences
Dr. Charles Severin
Assistant Dean, Admissions
Room 131, Biomed. Ed. Building
3435 Main Street
Buffalo, NY 14214
716-829-3466

State University of New York
at Stony Brook
School of Medicine
Health Sciences Center
Jack Fuhrer
Associate Dean/Director of
Admissions – Level 4
Room 147A
Stony Brook, NY 11794-8434
631-444-2113

State University of New York –
Upstate Medical Univeristy
College of Medicine
E. Gregory Keating, Ph.D.
Dean, Student Affairs
766 Irving Avenue
Syracuse, NY 13210
315-464-4570

NORTH CAROLINA

The Brody School of Medicine at
  East Carolina University
Dr. James G. Peden Jr.
Associate Dean for Admissions
Office of Admissions
600 Moye Blvd.
Greenville, NC 27834
252-816-2202

Duke University
  School of Medicine
Dr. Brenda E. Armstrong
Associate Dean, Director of
  Admissions
P.O. Box 3710
Durham, NC 27710
919-684-2985

University of North Carolina at
  Chapel Hill
  School of Medicine
Dr. Axalla Hoole
CB9500
Associate Dean – Admissions
121 MacNider Hall
Chapel Hill, NC 27599
919-962-8331

Wake Forrest University
  School of Medicine
Bowman Gray Campus
Dr. Lewis H. Nelson, III
Associate Dean for Admissions
Medical Center Boulevard
Winston-Salem, NC 27157-1090
336-716-4264

NORTH DAKOTA

University of North Dakota*
  School of Medicine and Health
  Sciences
Judy L. DeMers
Associate Dean, Student Affairs &
  Admissions
501 N. Columbia Road, Box 9037
Grand Forks, ND 58202-9037
701-777-4221

OHIO

Case Western Reserve University
  School of Medicine
Dr. Amy Henighan
Associate Dean for Admissions
Room E-308
10900 Euclid Avenue
Cleveland, OH 44106-4920
216-368-3450

University of Cincinnati
  College of Medicine
Dr. Laura Wexler
Associate Dean for Student Affairs
  and Admissions
P.O. Box 670552
Cincinnati, OH 45267-0552
513-558-7314

Medical College of Ohio
Dr. Mary Ann Myers
Associate Dean for Admissions
Mulford Library Bldg, Rm. 103
3045 Arlington Avenue
Toledo, OH 43614-5805
419-383-4229

Northeastern Ohio Universities
College of Medicine
Dr. Stephen Manuel
Director of Admissions
P.O. Box 95
4209 State Rt 44
Rootstown, OH 44272-0095
330-325-6270

Ohio State University
College of Medicine
Don Batisky, M.D.
Associate Dean of Admissions and
Student Records
Room 155E Meiling Hall
370 W. Ninth Avenue
Columbus, OH 43210-1238
614-292-7137

Ohio University
College of Osteopathic Medicine§
John Schriner
Director of Admissions
102 Grosvenor Hall
Athens, OH 45701-2979
740-593-4313

Wright State University
School of Medicine
Dr. Paul G. Carlson
Associate Dean for Admissions
P.O. Box 1751
Dayton, OH 45401
937-775-2934

OKLAHOMA

Oklahoma State University
College of Osteopathic Medicine§
Leah Haines
Assistant Director of Admissions
and Recruitment
1111 W. 17th Street
Tulsa, OK 74107
918-582-1972

University of Oklahoma
College of Medicine
Dotty Shaw Killam
Director for Admissions
BMSB – 374
P.O. Box 26901
Oklahoma City, OK 73190
405-271-2331

OREGON

Oregon Health & Science University
School of Medicine
Vicki Fields
Assistant Dean for Medical
Education
3181 SW Sam Jackson Park Road
Portland, OR 97239
503-494-2998

PENNSYLVANIA

Lake Erie College of Osteopathic
Medicine§
Elaine Morse
Admissions Coordinator
1858 W. Grandview Boulevard
Erie, PA 16509
814-866-6641

Jefferson Medical College
Dr. Clara Callahan
Vice Dean for Admissions
1015 Walnut Street, Suite 110
Philadelphia, PA 19107
215-955-6983

Drexel University
College of Medicine
Dr. Alan Tunkel
Assoc Dean of Admissions
2900 Queen Lane
Philadelphia, PA 19129
215-991-8202

Pennsylvania State University
  College of Medicine
Dr. Dwight Davis
Associate Dean of Student Affairs
  and Admissions
Suite H060
500 University Drive
P.O. Box 850
Hershey, PA 17033
717-531-8755

Philadelphia College of Osteopathic
  Medicine§
Carol Fox
Associate Vice President of
  Enrollment Management
4170 City Avenue
Philadelphia, PA 19131
215-871-6100

University of Pennsylvania
  School of Medicine
Gaye W. Sheffler
Director of Admissions
Office of Admissions/Financial Aid
Suite 100, Stemmler Hall
3450 Hamilton Walk
Philadelphia, PA 19104-6056
215-898-8001

University of Pittsburgh
  School of Medicine
Dr. Edward I. Curtiss
Associate Dean of Admissions
518 Scaife Hall
3550 Terrace Street
Pittsburgh, PA 15261
412-648-9891

Temple University
  School of Medicine
Audrey B. Uknis, M.D.
Associate Dean for Admissions
Suite 305 Student Faculty Center
3340 N. Broad Street
Philadelphia, PA 19140
215-707-3656

PUERTO RICO

Universidad Central del Caribe
  School of Medicine
Dr. Jose Ginel Rodriguez
Acting Dean of Medicine
Office of Admissions
P.O. Box 60-327
Bayamon, Puerto Rico 00960-6032
787-740-1611

Ponce School of Medicine
Dr. Carmen M. Mercado
Assistant Dean of Admissions
P.O. Box 7004
Ponce, Puerto Rico 00732-7004
787-840-2511

University of Puerto Rico
Medical Sciences Campus
Rosa Velez
Director of Admissions
P.O. Box 365067
San Juan, Puerto Rico 00936-5067
787-758-2525

RHODE ISLAND

Brown University
  School of Medicine*
Dr. Stephen R. Smith
Associate Dean for Medical
  Education
Box G-A212
97 Waterman Street
Providence, RI 02912-9706
401-863-2149

SOUTH CAROLINA

Medical University of South
   Carolina College of Medicine
Dr. Paul Underwood
Chair for Admissions
41 Bee Street
P.O. Box 250203
Charleston, SC 29425
843-792-3281

University of South Carolina
   School of Medicine
Dr. Richard Hoppmann
Office of Admission and
   Enrollment
Columbia, SC 29208
803-733-3325

SOUTH DAKOTA

University of South Dakota
   School of Medicine
Dr. Paul Bunger
Dean – Admissions
Lee Medical Building, Room 105
414 E. Clark Street
Vermillion, SD 57069-2390
605-677-5233

TENNESSEE

East Tennessee State University
   James H. Quillen College of
   Medicine
Edwin D. Taylor
Assistant Dean for Admissions
P.O. Box 70580
Johnson City, TN 37614-0580
423-439-2033

Meharry Medical College
   School of Medicine
Allen Mosley
Director/Admissions and Records
1005 D.B. Todd Boulevard
Nashville, TN 37208
615-327-6223

University of Tennessee
   Memphis College of Medicine
Dr. Hershel P. Wall
Associate Dean for Admissions and
   Student Affairs
710 Madison Avenue
Memphis, TN 38163-2166
901-448-5559

Vanderbilt University
   School of Medicine
Pat Sagen
Director of Admissions Committee
215 Light Hall
Nashville, TN 37232-0685
615-322-2145

TEXAS

Baylor College of Medicine
Dr. Lloyd Michaels
Dean of Admissions
Office of Admissions
One Baylor Plaza, Room N104
Houston, TX 77030
713-798-4842

Texas A&M University
   Health Sciences Center
   College of Medicine*
Filomeno G. Maldonado
Assistant Dean of Admissions
159 Reynolds Medical Bldg.
College Station, TX 77843-1114
979-845-7744

Texas College of Osteopathic
    Medicine[§]
Joel Daboub
Director Medical Student
    Admissions
3500 Camp Bowie Blvd.
Fort Worth, TX 76107
817-735-2204

Texas Tech University*
    Health Sciences Center
    School of Medicine
Dr. Bernell Dalley
Associate Dean of Education
3601 4th Street
Lubbock, TX 79430-6216
806-743-2297

University of Texas
    Southwestern Medical Center
    at Dallas
Dr. Scott Wright
Director of Admissions
5323 Harry Hines Boulevard
Dallas, TX 75390-9162
214-648-5617

University of Texas*
    Medical School at Galveston
Dr. Lauree Thomas
Associate Dean – Admissions and
    Student Affairs
301 University Blvd.
Galveston, TX 77555-1317
409-772-1442

University of Texas*
    Houston Medical School
Albert E. Gunn, Esq.
Associate Dean for Admissions
6431 Fannin
MSB 1.126
Houston, TX 77030
713-500-5116

University of Texas*
    Medical School at San Antonio
Dr. David J. Jones
Dean of Admissions
7703 Floyd Curl Drive
San Antonio, TX 78229-3900
210-567-2665

UTAH

University of Utah
    School of Medicine
Dr. Wayne Samuelson
Associate Dean, Admissions
30 North 1900 East #1C029
Salt Lake City, UT 84132
801-581-7498

VERMONT

University of Vermont
    College of Medicine
Tiffany Delaney
Associate Director for Admissions
E-215 Given Building
89 Beaumont Avenue
Burlington, VT 05405-0068
802-656-2154

VIRGINIA

Eastern Virginia Medical School
    of the Medical College of
    Hampton Roads
Susan L. Castora
Director of Admissions
700 West Onley Road
Norfolk, VA 23507
757-446-5812

Edward Via Virginia College of
  Osteopathic Medicine§
Megan Settle
Director of Admissions
2265 Kraft Drive
Blacksburg, VA 24060
540-231-4000

Virginia Commonwealth University
  Medical College of Virginia
  School of Medicine
Cynthia M. Heldberg
Assoc. Dean for Admissions
MCV Station, Box 980565
Richmond, VA 23298-0565
804-828-9629

University of Virginia
  School of Medicine
Dr. Beth A. Bailey
Director of Admissions
Admissions Office, Box 800725
Charlotteville, VA 22908
434-924-5571

WASHINGTON

University of Washington
  School of Medicine
Dr. Werner E. Sampson
Dean for Admissions
Health Sciences Center A-300
Box 356340
Seattle, WA 98195-6340
206-543-7212

WEST VIRGINIA

Marshall University
  School of Medicine
Cynthia A. Warren
Assistant Dean of Admissions
1600 Medical Center Drive
Suite 3400
Huntington, WV 25701-3655
304-691-1738

West Virginia School of
  Osteopathic Medicine§
Donna Varney
Director of Admissions
400 North Lee Street
Lewisburg, WV 24901
800-356-7836

West Virginia University
  School of Medicine
Dr. David Morgan
Director of Admissions Committee
P.O. Box 9111
Morgantown, WV 26506-9111
304-293-2408

WISCONSIN

Medical College of Wisconsin
Michael Istwan
Director of Admissions
8701 Watertown Plank Road
Miiwaukee, WI 53226
414-456-8246

University of Wisconsin
  Medical School
Lucy J. Wall
Assistant Dean of Admissions
Health Sciences Learning Center
Room 2138
750 Highland Avenue
Madison, WI 53705
608-263-4925

* Denotes non-AMCAS allopathic
medical school

§ Denotes osteopathic medical
school

Personal Notes

Personal Notes

Personal Notes

Personal Notes